Facial Yoga Exercise Guide for Beginners

Understanding the Benefits of Facial Yoga Exercise

By

Artair Gilroy

Table of Contents

CHAPTER 1

Introduction to Face Yoga

1.1 What is Face Yoga?

Face yoga, also known as facial yoga or facial exercises, is a natural, non-invasive approach to facial rejuvenation and wellness. Just as yoga exercises benefit the body's muscles and promote overall physical health, face yoga targets the muscles of the face, neck, and jaw to tone, lift, and rejuvenate the appearance of the skin. It involves a series of specific movements, poses, and techniques designed to stimulate circulation, improve muscle tone, and reduce tension in the facial muscles.

Unlike surgical or injectable procedures, face yoga is completely natural and relies on the body's innate ability to heal and regenerate. By engaging in regular face yoga practices, individuals can potentially achieve a more youthful and radiant appearance without the risks or side effects associated with invasive procedures. Face yoga is often regarded as a holistic approach to skincare, as it not only addresses the physical aspects of facial aging but also promotes relaxation, mindfulness, and overall well-being.

The practice of face yoga draws inspiration from various disciplines, including traditional yoga, acupressure, facial massage, and mindfulness techniques. While the concept of facial exercises has been around for centuries in some form, the modern popularity of face yoga can be attributed to its accessibility and effectiveness in promoting facial health and beauty.

One of the fundamental principles of face yoga is the recognition of the interconnectedness between the facial muscles, skin, and underlying structures. Just as tension and stress in the body can manifest as physical discomfort or pain, repetitive facial expressions, poor posture, and lifestyle factors can contribute to the development of wrinkles, sagging skin, and other signs of aging on the face.

By practicing face yoga regularly, individuals can learn to release tension, increase circulation, and improve the overall health and appearance of their facial muscles and skin. Additionally, face yoga encourages mindfulness and self-awareness, allowing practitioners to cultivate a deeper connection with their bodies and emotions.

face yoga is a holistic practice that combines physical exercises, mindfulness techniques, and self-care practices to promote facial rejuvenation, wellness, and overall vitality. It offers a natural alternative to invasive cosmetic procedures and empowers individuals to take control of their facial health and beauty in a safe and sustainable way.

1.2 Benefits of Face Yoga

Face yoga offers a wide range of benefits that extend beyond just improving the appearance of the face. Here are some of the key benefits:

1. Enhanced Muscle Tone: Just like traditional yoga strengthens and tones muscles throughout the body, face yoga exercises target the muscles of the face, neck, and jaw, helping to improve their tone and firmness. This can result in a more lifted and sculpted appearance, reducing the appearance of sagging skin and wrinkles.

2. Increased Circulation: The gentle massaging and stretching motions involved in face yoga help to stimulate blood flow to the facial muscles and skin. Improved circulation can promote a healthy complexion by delivering oxygen and nutrients to the skin cells, while also aiding in the removal of toxins and waste products.

3. Reduced Tension and Stress: The face is a common area where people hold tension, especially in the jaw,

forehead, and around the eyes. Face yoga techniques, such as relaxation exercises and acupressure points, can help to release tension and alleviate stress in these areas. This can result in a more relaxed and youthful appearance, as well as reduced discomfort or pain associated with tension headaches or temporomandibular joint (TMJ) dysfunction.

4. Prevention of Premature Aging: By strengthening and toning the facial muscles, face yoga can help to prevent and reduce the appearance of common signs of aging, such as fine lines, wrinkles, and sagging skin. Regular practice of face yoga exercises can also promote collagen production, which contributes to the skin's elasticity and firmness, helping to maintain a youthful appearance over time.

5. Improved Facial Symmetry and Balance: Face yoga exercises often involve movements that target both

sides of the face equally, helping to improve symmetry and balance in facial features. This can be particularly beneficial for individuals who have asymmetrical features or who wish to enhance their facial harmony and proportion.

6. Mind-Body Connection: Like traditional yoga, face yoga emphasizes the connection between the mind and body. By practicing mindfulness techniques and focusing on the sensations in the face and body during exercises, practitioners can cultivate a greater sense of self-awareness and inner peace. This holistic approach to facial health and beauty can contribute to overall well-being and emotional balance.

7. Cost-Effective and Non-Invasive: Unlike surgical or injectable procedures, face yoga requires no special equipment or expensive products. It can be practiced anywhere, anytime, making it a convenient and cost-effective

alternative for those seeking natural methods of facial rejuvenation. Additionally, face yoga carries minimal risk of side effects or complications, making it a safe and non-invasive option for individuals of all ages and skin types.

The benefits of face yoga extend beyond just improving the appearance of the face, offering holistic wellness benefits for both the body and mind. By incorporating face yoga into their regular self-care routine, individuals can experience improved facial health, enhanced relaxation, and a greater sense of overall vitality and well-being.

CHAPTER 2

Understanding Facial Muscles

2.1 Anatomy of the Face

To understand face yoga and its effects, it's essential to have a basic understanding of the anatomy of the face. The human face is a complex structure composed of numerous muscles, bones, and soft tissues that work together to facilitate facial expressions, speech, eating, and other essential functions. Here's an overview of the key components of facial anatomy:

1. **Skin**: The outermost layer of the face, the skin, serves as a protective barrier against external factors such as sunlight, pollutants, and microorganisms. It contains hair follicles, sweat glands, and

sebaceous glands, which help regulate temperature and moisture levels.

2. **Muscles**: The face contains over 40 individual muscles responsible for producing a wide range of facial expressions. These muscles are divided into two main groups: superficial and deep muscles.

    - **Superficial Muscles**: These muscles are located closer to the skin's surface and are primarily responsible for creating visible facial expressions. Examples include the orbicularis oculi (around the eyes), orbicularis oris (around the mouth), and frontalis (forehead).

    - **Deep Muscles**: Situated deeper within the face, these muscles play a role in stabilizing facial movements and supporting the structure of the face. Examples include the masseter (jaw), buccinator (cheeks), and platysma (neck).

3. **Facial Bones**: The facial skeleton
    provides the framework for the face and
    serves as attachment points for the
    muscles. Key facial bones include the
    mandible (lower jaw), maxilla (upper
    jaw), zygomatic bones (cheekbones),
    and frontal bone (forehead).

4. **Fat Deposits**: Beneath the skin and
    muscles, the face contains various fat
    deposits that contribute to its volume and
    shape. These fat pads provide support
    and cushioning, giving the face its
    youthful contours.

5. **Nerves and Blood Vessels**: The face is
    richly supplied with nerves and blood
    vessels that supply oxygen, nutrients,
    and sensory information to the tissues.
    Facial nerves control muscle movements
    and transmit sensory signals such as
    touch, pain, and temperature.

Understanding the anatomy of the face is
essential for practicing face yoga effectively.
By targeting specific muscles and areas of
the face through exercise and massage
techniques, individuals can strengthen

muscles, improve circulation, and promote overall facial health and vitality. Additionally, awareness of facial anatomy can help practitioners identify areas of tension or imbalance and tailor their practice to address specific concerns or goals.

2.2 Common Facial Muscle Groups

Understanding the common facial muscle groups is crucial for effectively practicing face yoga and targeting specific areas for rejuvenation and relaxation. Here are some of the key muscle groups in the face:

1. **Orbicularis Oculi**: This muscle surrounds the eye and is responsible for closing the eyelids. It consists of two parts: the orbital part, which closes the eyelids gently, and the palpebral part, which provides a stronger closure. Strengthening and toning the orbicularis oculi muscles can help reduce the appearance of crow's feet and eye bags.

2. **Orbicularis Oris**: Encircling the
    mouth, the orbicularis oris muscle
    controls lip movements, including
    puckering, smiling, and kissing.
    Strengthening this muscle group can
    enhance lip definition and reduce the
    appearance of fine lines around the
    mouth.

3. **Frontalis**: Located in the forehead
    region, the frontalis muscle is
    responsible for raising the eyebrows
    and creating forehead wrinkles when
    expressing surprise or curiosity. By
    practicing exercises to tone and relax
    the frontalis, individuals can reduce
    tension in the forehead and minimize
    the appearance of horizontal lines.

4. **Zygomaticus Major and Minor**:
    These muscles extend from the
    cheekbones to the corners of the
    mouth and are involved in smiling
    and lifting the corners of the lips.
    Strengthening the zygomaticus
    muscles can help elevate the cheeks,
    improve facial symmetry, and

diminish the appearance of nasolabial folds (smile lines).

5. **Buccinator**: The buccinator muscle is located in the cheeks and is responsible for compressing the cheeks inward during activities such as blowing, sucking, and chewing. Exercises targeting the buccinator can help enhance cheek definition and promote a more sculpted appearance.

6. **Masseter**: Situated along the jawline, the masseter muscle is one of the primary muscles involved in chewing and jaw movement. Tension or overuse of the masseter can contribute to jaw pain, teeth grinding, and a squared jawline. Masseter exercises can help relieve tension and sculpt the jawline for a more defined appearance.

7. **Platysma**: Extending from the lower jaw to the collarbone and chest, the platysma muscle is involved in movements such as swallowing,

speaking, and facial expressions of tension or surprise. Strengthening and toning the platysma can help improve the appearance of the neck and jawline by reducing sagging and enhancing muscle definition.

These common facial muscle groups allows individuals to tailor their face yoga practice to target specific areas of concern and achieve desired aesthetic outcomes. By engaging in targeted exercises and techniques, practitioners can strengthen facial muscles, improve circulation, and promote overall facial health and vitality. Additionally, regular face yoga practice can help reduce tension, stress, and signs of aging, resulting in a more relaxed, youthful, and radiant appearance.

2.3 How Face Yoga Targets Muscles

Face yoga utilizes a variety of techniques to target and engage the muscles of the face, neck, and jaw. By incorporating specific exercises, stretches, and massage techniques, face yoga aims to strengthen, tone, and rejuvenate these muscles, resulting in improved facial appearance and overall well-being. Here's how face yoga effectively targets facial muscles:

1. **Isometric Contractions**: Face yoga exercises often involve isometric contractions, which means contracting and holding specific facial muscles without moving the surrounding skin. This helps to strengthen and tone the muscles without causing unnecessary strain on the skin or joints. For example, exercises like the "forehead smoother" involve lifting the eyebrows while simultaneously pressing them down with the fingertips, engaging the frontalis muscle to reduce forehead wrinkles.

2. **Resistance Training**: Some face yoga exercises incorporate resistance training techniques to challenge and strengthen the facial muscles. This can involve using the hands or

fingers to provide resistance against facial movements, such as pressing against the cheeks while smiling to engage the zygomaticus muscles. Resistance training helps to build muscle strength and endurance, leading to improved muscle tone and definition over time.

3. **Dynamic Movements**: Face yoga incorporates dynamic movements and stretches to increase flexibility and range of motion in the facial muscles. These movements help to release tension, improve circulation, and promote relaxation in the muscles and surrounding tissues. For example, exercises like the "lion face" involve stretching the facial muscles while making exaggerated facial expressions, helping to release tightness and stiffness.

4. **Facial Massage**: Massage techniques are often integrated into face yoga routines to stimulate circulation, promote lymphatic drainage, and release tension in the

facial muscles. Massaging the face with gentle, upward strokes helps to relax the muscles, reduce puffiness, and improve the absorption of skincare products. Additionally, acupressure points may be targeted during facial massage to enhance energy flow and promote overall facial harmony.

5. **Breathing Techniques**: Mindful breathing techniques are an essential aspect of face yoga, as they help to increase oxygenation and relaxation in the facial muscles. Deep breathing exercises encourage relaxation of the facial muscles and promote a sense of calmness and well-being. Practitioners may incorporate breath awareness into their face yoga practice to enhance the mind-body connection and optimize the benefits of the exercises.

face yoga targets muscles through a combination of isometric contractions, resistance training, dynamic movements, facial massage, and breathing techniques.

By engaging in regular practice, individuals can strengthen and tone their facial muscles, improve circulation, and achieve a more youthful, radiant appearance. Additionally, face yoga promotes relaxation, stress relief, and overall facial health, making it a holistic approach to facial rejuvenation and wellness.

CHAPTER 3

Basic Face Yoga Techniques

3.1 Relaxation and Warm-Up Exercises

Before diving into more intensive face yoga exercises, it's essential to start with relaxation and warm-up techniques to prepare the facial muscles and promote a sense of calmness and receptivity. These gentle exercises help to release tension, increase circulation, and create a foundation for the rest of your practice. Here are some basic relaxation and warm-up exercises for the face:

1. **Deep Breathing**: Begin by finding a comfortable seated or standing position with your spine straight and

shoulders relaxed. Close your eyes and take a few deep breaths in through your nose, allowing your abdomen to expand fully. Then exhale slowly through your mouth, releasing any tension or stress with each breath. Continue deep breathing for several rounds, focusing on the sensation of the breath as it enters and leaves your body.

2. **Neck Rolls**: Gently drop your chin towards your chest and roll your head slowly from side to side, bringing your right ear towards your right shoulder and then your left ear towards your left shoulder. Repeat this movement several times, allowing your neck muscles to relax and release any tension. Avoid rolling your head backward to prevent strain on the neck muscles.

3. **Shoulder Shrugs**: Lift your shoulders towards your ears as you inhale deeply, feeling the tension in your shoulders. Hold for a moment, then exhale as you release your

shoulders down and back, letting go of any tightness or stress. Repeat this shoulder shrugging motion several times, allowing your shoulders to become more relaxed with each repetition.

4. **Facial Massage**: Using your fingertips, gently massage your temples in circular motions, moving towards your hairline. Then, massage your jawline, starting from the chin and moving towards the ears. Finally, massage your forehead with upward strokes, starting from the eyebrows and moving towards the hairline. This facial massage helps to stimulate circulation, release tension, and promote relaxation in the facial muscles.

5. **Cheek Puffing**: Inhale deeply through your nose and puff out your cheeks as you hold the breath for a few seconds. Then, exhale slowly through your mouth, feeling the air gently escape from your cheeks. Repeat this cheek puffing exercise

several times, noticing the sensation of expansion and relaxation in the cheeks and facial muscles.

6. **Eye Relaxation**: Close your eyes gently and place your fingertips lightly over your eyelids. Apply gentle pressure to the eyelids, feeling the warmth of your fingertips and the gentle pressure against your eyes. Hold for a few seconds, then release the pressure and allow your eyes to rest naturally. This eye relaxation exercise helps to soothe tired eyes and reduce strain from screen time or extended periods of concentration.

Incorporating these relaxation and warm-up exercises into your face yoga routine, you can prepare your facial muscles and mind for the more intensive exercises to follow. These gentle techniques promote relaxation, reduce tension, and create a sense of ease and openness in the face, allowing you to fully benefit from your face yoga practice.

3.2 Facial Massage Techniques

Facial massage is a key component of face yoga, helping to stimulate circulation, release tension, and promote relaxation in the facial muscles and skin. Incorporating massage techniques into your face yoga routine can enhance the effectiveness of your practice and contribute to a more youthful, radiant appearance. Here are some facial massage techniques to try:

1. **Forehead Massage**: Start by applying a small amount of facial oil or moisturizer to your fingertips. Using gentle upward strokes, massage your forehead from the eyebrows to the hairline. Use circular motions to massage the temples, applying light pressure to release tension. Continue massaging the

forehead for several minutes, focusing on areas of tightness or discomfort.

2. **Eye Massage**: Using your index and middle fingers, gently massage the area around your eyes in circular motions. Start from the inner corners of the eyes and move outwards towards the temples, applying light pressure. Be careful not to tug or pull on the delicate skin around the eyes. Repeat this massage technique several times to reduce puffiness and promote lymphatic drainage.

3. **Cheek Massage**: With your fingertips, massage your cheeks using upward and outward strokes. Start from the center of your face and move towards the ears, applying gentle pressure to stimulate circulation and promote collagen production. You can also use a jade roller or gua sha tool to enhance the massage and reduce tension in the cheeks.

4. **Jawline Massage**: Place your fingertips on your jawline and massage in small circular motions, moving from the chin towards the ears. Apply firm but gentle pressure to release tension in the jaw muscles and improve definition along the jawline. You can also use your knuckles to massage the jawline in an upward motion for added stimulation.

5. **Neck Massage**: Extend the massage down to the neck, using your fingertips to massage the muscles on either side of the neck. Start from the base of the neck and work your way up towards the jawline, applying gentle pressure to release tension and improve circulation. You can also incorporate kneading or tapping motions to further relax the neck muscles.

6. **Acupressure Points**: Explore acupressure points on the face and neck to target specific areas of tension or discomfort. For example,

pressing gently on the acupressure point between the eyebrows (known as the third eye point) can help relieve headaches and promote relaxation. Similarly, applying pressure to the acupressure points along the jawline can help reduce jaw tension and promote overall facial harmony.

7. **Finish with Relaxation**: After completing your facial massage, take a moment to relax and let go of any remaining tension in the face and body. Close your eyes and take a few deep breaths, allowing yourself to fully experience the benefits of the massage. Notice any sensations or feelings of relaxation that arise, and take this time to cultivate a sense of inner peace and well-being.

These facial massage techniques into your face yoga routine, you can enhance circulation, release tension, and promote a more youthful, radiant appearance. Experiment with different massage movements and techniques to find what works best for your unique facial needs and preferences. With regular practice, facial massage can become a rejuvenating and enjoyable part of your self-care routine.

3.3 Breathing Techniques for Face Yoga

Breathing techniques play a vital role in face yoga, helping to promote relaxation, mindfulness, and overall well-being. By incorporating conscious breathing into your face yoga practice, you can enhance the benefits of the exercises and deepen your connection with your body and breath. Here are some breathing techniques to try during your face yoga sessions:

1. **Deep Belly Breathing**: Start by finding a comfortable seated or standing position with your spine straight and shoulders relaxed. Place one hand on your abdomen, just below your rib cage, and the other hand on your chest. Inhale deeply through your nose, allowing your

abdomen to expand fully as you fill your lungs with air. Feel your diaphragm move downward and your belly rise against your hand. Exhale slowly through your mouth, allowing your abdomen to contract as you release the breath. Continue deep belly breathing for several rounds, focusing on the sensation of the breath moving in and out of your body.

2. **Alternate Nostril Breathing**: Sit in a comfortable position with your spine straight and shoulders relaxed. Place your left hand on your left knee, palm facing upward. Bring your right hand up to your nose, with your index and middle fingers resting between your eyebrows and your thumb resting on your right nostril. Close your right nostril with your thumb and inhale deeply through your left nostril. Close your left nostril with your ring finger and release your thumb from your right nostril. Exhale fully through your

right nostril. Inhale deeply through your right nostril. Close your right nostril with your thumb and release your ring finger from your left nostril. Exhale fully through your left nostril. Continue alternating nostrils for several rounds, maintaining a smooth and steady breath.

3. **Sitali (Cooling Breath)**: Sit in a comfortable position with your spine straight and shoulders relaxed. Curl your tongue into a tube shape, sticking it slightly out of your mouth. Inhale deeply through your curled tongue, feeling the cool air entering your mouth and throat. Close your mouth and exhale slowly through your nose, feeling the warm air leaving your body. If you're unable to curl your tongue, you can purse your lips and sip the air in through the teeth instead. Repeat this cooling breath for several rounds, focusing on the sensation of coolness on the inhale and warmth on the exhale.

4. **Lion's Breath (Simhasana Pranayama)**: Sit in a comfortable position with your spine straight and shoulders relaxed. Place your hands on your knees or thighs, with your fingers spread wide. Inhale deeply through your nose, filling your lungs with air. As you exhale forcefully through your mouth, open your mouth wide, stick out your tongue, and roar like a lion, making a "ha" sound. Simultaneously, stretch your eyes wide, gaze upward, and contract the muscles of your face, including the forehead, cheeks, and jaw. Repeat this lion's breath for several rounds, allowing yourself to release tension and express yourself freely.

5. **Counted Breathing**: Sit in a comfortable position with your spine straight and shoulders relaxed. Close your eyes and take a few deep breaths to center yourself. Inhale deeply through your nose for a count of four seconds, feeling the breath fill your lungs completely. Hold your

breath at the top of the inhale for a count of four seconds, allowing yourself to fully absorb the breath. Exhale slowly and steadily through your nose for a count of six seconds, releasing any tension or stress with each breath. Pause briefly at the bottom of the exhale for a count of two seconds before beginning the next breath cycle. Continue this counted breathing pattern for several minutes, focusing on the rhythm of your breath and the sensations in your body.

These breathing techniques into your face yoga practice, you can enhance relaxation, promote mindfulness, and deepen your connection with your body and breath. Experiment with different techniques to find what works best for you, and remember to listen to your body and adjust your practice as needed. With regular practice, breathing techniques can become a powerful tool for promoting overall well-being and vitality.

CHAPTER 4

Beginner Face Yoga Exercises

4.1 Forehead Smoother

This exercise aims to relax and smooth the muscles of the forehead, reducing tension and minimizing the appearance of lines and wrinkles.

Instructions:

1. Begin by sitting comfortably with your spine straight and shoulders relaxed.

2. Place your fingertips lightly on your forehead, just above your eyebrows.

3. Gently press your fingertips into your forehead, applying light pressure.

4. While keeping your fingertips in place, try to raise your eyebrows as high as possible.

5. Hold this raised position for a few seconds, feeling the stretch in your forehead muscles.

6. Relax and release the tension in your forehead, allowing your eyebrows to return to their natural position.

7. Repeat this movement 5-10 times, focusing on smooth, controlled movements and deep breathing throughout the exercise.

Benefits:

- Relaxes and tones the muscles of the forehead.

- Helps to reduce tension and stress in the forehead area.

- Improves circulation and promotes a more youthful appearance.

4.2 Cheek Plumper

This exercise focuses on toning and firming the muscles of the cheeks, promoting a more lifted and youthful appearance.

Instructions:

1. Sit or stand in a comfortable position with your spine straight and shoulders relaxed.

2. Begin by smiling widely, showing your teeth.

3. While maintaining the smile, press the fingertips of both hands firmly against the cheeks.

4. Use your fingertips to lift the cheeks upward towards the eyes, resisting the pressure with the muscles of your cheeks.

5. Hold this lifted position for 5-10 seconds, feeling the muscles of your cheeks working.

6. Relax and release the pressure, allowing your cheeks to return to their natural position.

7. Repeat this exercise 5-10 times, focusing on smooth, controlled movements and deep breathing throughout.

Benefits:

- Strengthens and tones the muscles of the cheeks, promoting a more lifted appearance.

- Improves circulation and enhances the natural contour of the cheeks.

- Reduces the appearance of sagging or drooping in the cheek area.

- Provides a natural alternative to invasive procedures such as cheek fillers or implants.

The cheek plumper exercise into your face yoga routine, you can enhance the definition and contour of your cheeks, promoting a more youthful and radiant appearance over time. Consistent practice and patience are key to achieving the desired results.

4.3 Jawline Definition

This exercise targets the muscles along the jawline, helping to strengthen and define the jawline for a more sculpted appearance.

Instructions:

1. Sit or stand in a comfortable position with your spine straight and shoulders relaxed.

2. Begin by tilting your head slightly back, lifting your chin towards the ceiling.

3. Close your lips together and press your tongue firmly against the roof of your mouth.

4. Slowly and steadily, begin to open and close your mouth, maintaining the pressure of your tongue against the roof of your mouth throughout the movement.

5. As you open your mouth, imagine extending your jawline forward, as if you were trying to touch your chin to your chest.

6. As you close your mouth, imagine drawing your chin back towards your throat, feeling the muscles of your jaw working.

7. Repeat this movement 10-15 times, focusing on smooth, controlled movements and maintaining the pressure of your tongue against the roof of your mouth.

Benefits:

- Strengthens and tones the muscles along the jawline, promoting a more defined appearance.

- Helps to reduce sagging or drooping in the jawline area.

- Improves circulation and lymphatic drainage, reducing puffiness and promoting a more sculpted contour.

- Provides a natural alternative to invasive procedures such as jawline fillers or implants.

The jawline definition exercise into your face yoga routine to enhance the definition and contour of your jawline, promoting a more youthful and sculpted appearance over time. Consistent practice and patience are essential for achieving the desired results.

CHAPTER 5

Creating a Face Yoga Routine

5.1 Designing Your Routine

Designing a personalized face yoga routine allows you to target specific areas of concern and incorporate exercises that resonate with your needs and preferences. Here are some steps to help you design an effective face yoga routine:

1. **Identify Your Goals**: Determine what you hope to achieve through face yoga. Whether you want to reduce wrinkles, tone specific facial muscles, improve circulation, or promote relaxation, clarifying your

goals will guide the selection of exercises for your routine.

2. **Assess Your Current Needs**: Take note of any areas of tension, stiffness, or imbalance in your face and neck. Consider factors such as stress levels, posture habits, and lifestyle factors that may impact the health and appearance of your skin and muscles.

3. **Select Targeted Exercises**: Choose a variety of face yoga exercises that target your specific goals and address areas of concern. Focus on exercises that strengthen, tone, and relax the muscles of the face, neck, and jaw. Include a mix of exercises for different muscle groups, such as the forehead, eyes, cheeks, jawline, and neck.

4. **Consider Your Schedule**: Determine how much time you can dedicate to your face yoga routine each day or week. Aim for consistency by selecting exercises

that fit within your schedule and are realistic to maintain over time. Even short daily sessions can yield noticeable results with regular practice.

5. **Sequence Your Exercises**: Arrange your selected exercises in a logical sequence that flows smoothly from one movement to the next. Begin with relaxation and warm-up exercises to prepare your muscles and mind for the practice. Progress to targeted exercises that address your specific goals, alternating between strengthening, toning, and stretching movements. Conclude your routine with relaxation and breathing techniques to promote a sense of calmness and integration.

6. **Practice Mindfulness and Breath Awareness**: Throughout your face yoga routine, cultivate mindfulness and awareness of your breath. Focus on the sensations in your body as you perform each exercise, noticing areas of tension or release. Pay

attention to your breath, taking slow,
deep breaths to oxygenate your
muscles and promote relaxation.

7. **Listen to Your Body**: Honor your
   body's feedback and adjust your
   routine as needed to accommodate
   any discomfort or limitations. Avoid
   forcing or straining your muscles and
   modify exercises as necessary to suit
   your individual needs and abilities.

8. **Track Your Progress**: Keep track
   of your progress by documenting
   changes in your facial appearance,
   muscle tone, and overall well-being
   over time. Take photos before
   starting your routine and periodically
   throughout your practice to monitor
   improvements. Notice any changes
   in the way your face feels and how
   you perceive yourself.

Following these steps and designing a
personalized face yoga routine, you can
tailor your practice to meet your specific
goals and preferences. Consistent practice
and patience are key to achieving lasting

results, so commit to integrating face yoga into your daily self-care routine for optimal benefits.

5.2 Setting Realistic Goals

When setting goals for your face yoga practice, it's essential to be realistic and mindful of what you hope to achieve. Here are some tips for setting achievable goals:

1. **Be Specific**: Clearly define your goals and objectives for practicing face yoga. Whether you aim to reduce wrinkles, tone facial muscles, improve circulation, or promote relaxation, specificity helps you focus your efforts and track your progress more effectively.

2. **Break It Down**: Break larger goals into smaller, more manageable milestones. For example, if your goal is to reduce forehead wrinkles, you might start by focusing on relaxation techniques and gradually incorporate

targeted exercises to strengthen and tone the forehead muscles over time.

3. **Set Measurable Targets**: Establish measurable targets to gauge your progress and success. This could involve tracking changes in your facial appearance, muscle tone, or flexibility over time. Consider taking photos or keeping a journal to document your journey and celebrate your achievements along the way.

4. **Be Realistic**: Set goals that are attainable within your current circumstances and capabilities. Consider factors such as your age, lifestyle, and commitment level when determining what is realistic for you. Avoid setting overly ambitious goals that may lead to frustration or disappointment.

5. **Focus on Process Goals**: Instead of solely focusing on outcomes, emphasize the process of practicing face yoga regularly. Set goals related to consistency, such as committing to

practicing a certain number of times per week or incorporating face yoga into your daily self-care routine. Consistent practice is key to achieving lasting results.

6. **Stay Flexible**: Be flexible and adaptable in your goal-setting approach. Allow yourself to adjust your goals as needed based on your progress, preferences, and changing circumstances. Stay open to exploring new techniques and exercises that resonate with you and support your overall well-being.

7. **Celebrate Progress**: Celebrate your progress and accomplishments along the way, no matter how small they may seem. Acknowledge your efforts and the positive changes you've experienced through your face yoga practice. Celebrating milestones can boost motivation and reinforce your commitment to your goals.

Setting realistic goals for your face yoga practice and staying focused on the process, you can cultivate a sustainable and fulfilling self-care routine that supports your overall health and well-being.

5.3 Integrating Face Yoga into Your Daily Life

Integrating face yoga into your daily life can be simple and rewarding, providing numerous benefits for your physical and mental well-being. Here are some tips for incorporating face yoga into your daily routine:

1. **Establish a Regular Practice Time**: Choose a consistent time each day to practice face yoga, such as in the morning before starting your day or in the evening as part of your bedtime routine. Consistency is key to forming a habit, so find a time that works best for you and stick to it.

2. **Start Small**: Begin with a few minutes of face yoga each day and

gradually increase the duration and intensity of your practice over time. Even a short daily practice can yield noticeable benefits for your facial muscles and skin.

3. **Integrate Face Yoga into Daily Activities**: Incorporate face yoga exercises into everyday activities, such as while watching TV, sitting at your desk, or during your skincare routine. Multi-tasking allows you to maximize your time and efficiency while still reaping the benefits of face yoga.

4. **Set Reminders**: Use reminders and cues to prompt you to practice face yoga throughout the day. Set alarms on your phone, place sticky notes in visible locations, or link your practice to existing habits or routines to help you stay on track.

5. **Practice Mindfulness**: Approach your face yoga practice with mindfulness and intention, focusing on the present moment and the

sensations in your body. Cultivate awareness of your breath, movements, and thoughts as you perform each exercise, allowing yourself to fully experience the benefits of your practice.

6. **Stay Flexible**: Be flexible and adaptable in your approach to practicing face yoga. If you miss a day or find it challenging to stick to your routine, don't be too hard on yourself. Instead, acknowledge any obstacles or setbacks and make adjustments as needed to maintain consistency over the long term.

7. **Make it Enjoyable**: Find ways to make your face yoga practice enjoyable and rewarding. Experiment with different exercises, techniques, and environments to keep your practice fresh and engaging. Listen to relaxing music, diffuse essential oils, or practice in front of a mirror to enhance your experience.

Integrating face yoga into your daily life in a sustainable and enjoyable way, you can experience the transformative benefits of this practice and enhance your overall health and well-being. Consistency, mindfulness, and self-care are key to cultivating a fulfilling face yoga routine that supports your unique needs and goals.

CHAPTER 6

Advanced Tips and Practices

6.1 Progressing Beyond Beginner Exercises

As you become more familiar with face yoga and build strength and flexibility in your facial muscles, you may want to incorporate more advanced techniques and practices into your routine. Here are some tips for progressing beyond beginner exercises:

1. **Gradually Increase Intensity**: Start by gradually increasing the intensity or duration of your existing

exercises. For example, you can hold each pose for a longer period or increase the number of repetitions to challenge your muscles further. Listen to your body and avoid overexertion by progressing at a pace that feels comfortable for you.

2. **Experiment with Variations**: Explore variations of familiar exercises to target different muscle groups and add variety to your routine. For example, you can modify the angle or direction of your movements, incorporate props such as resistance bands or exercise balls, or combine exercises to create more dynamic sequences.

3. **Focus on Muscle Isolation**: Practice isolating specific muscle groups to enhance precision and effectiveness in your exercises. Pay attention to the subtle nuances of each movement and concentrate on engaging the targeted muscles while minimizing tension in surrounding areas. This approach can help you develop

greater control and awareness of your facial muscles.

4. **Incorporate Resistance Training**: Integrate resistance training techniques into your face yoga practice to further challenge your muscles and stimulate growth. You can use your hands, fingers, or specialized tools such as facial rollers, gua sha stones, or facial exercise devices to provide resistance against your movements. Gradually increase the resistance over time as your muscles adapt and become stronger.

5. **Explore Advanced Breathing Techniques**: Experiment with advanced breathing techniques to deepen your practice and enhance relaxation. Techniques such as Kapalabhati (skull-shining breath), Bhramari (humming bee breath), or Nadi Shodhana (alternate nostril breathing) can help to purify the mind, calm the nervous system, and promote balance and harmony in the

body. Practice these techniques mindfully and gradually increase the duration and intensity as you become more proficient.

6. **Combine Face Yoga with Other Modalities**: Combine face yoga with other complementary practices such as yoga, meditation, mindfulness, or facial massage to create a holistic approach to facial rejuvenation and wellness. Experiment with integrating different modalities into your routine to address specific needs or goals and enhance the overall effectiveness of your practice.

7. **Seek Guidance from a Qualified Instructor**: Consider seeking guidance from a qualified face yoga instructor or practitioner who can provide personalized instruction, feedback, and guidance based on your individual needs and goals. A skilled instructor can offer insights, corrections, and modifications to

help you progress safely and effectively in your practice.

Progressing beyond beginner exercises and incorporating more advanced techniques and practices into your face yoga routine, you can continue to challenge yourself, deepen your practice, and achieve greater results in terms of muscle tone, facial rejuvenation, and overall well-being. Remember to listen to your body, practice with mindfulness, and enjoy the journey of self-discovery and transformation.

6.2 Fine-Tuning Technique and Form

Fine-tuning your technique and form in face yoga can significantly enhance the effectiveness of your practice and minimize the risk of injury. Here are some tips for refining your technique and form:

1. **Focus on Alignment**: Pay attention to your body's alignment and positioning during each exercise. Maintain a neutral spine, relaxed

shoulders, and engaged core to support stability and proper muscle activation. Avoid overarching or rounding your back and keep your head in a neutral position to avoid strain on the neck and spine.

2. **Mindful Muscle Engagement**: Cultivate awareness of the muscles you're targeting in each exercise and focus on engaging them mindfully. Concentrate on isolating and activating the specific muscle groups relevant to the exercise while minimizing tension in surrounding areas. Visualize the muscles contracting and releasing with each movement to enhance precision and effectiveness.

3. **Controlled Movement**: Perform each exercise with controlled and deliberate movements, avoiding jerky or erratic motions. Move slowly and smoothly through the full range of motion, maintaining tension in the muscles throughout the movement. Emphasize quality over

quantity, prioritizing proper form and technique over speed or intensity.

4. **Breath Awareness**: Coordinate your breath with your movements to enhance fluidity, relaxation, and mindfulness in your practice. Inhale deeply during the preparatory phase of the movement, and exhale slowly and steadily as you perform the action. Use your breath to facilitate relaxation, deepen stretches, and enhance muscle engagement.

5. **Modify as Needed**: Listen to your body's feedback and modify exercises as needed to accommodate any discomfort or limitations. Use props such as pillows, blocks, or straps to support your body and adapt exercises to suit your individual needs and abilities. Honor your body's boundaries and avoid pushing through pain or discomfort.

6. **Seek Feedback**: Consider seeking feedback from a qualified face yoga

instructor or practitioner who can provide guidance, corrections, and adjustments to refine your technique and form. A skilled instructor can offer insights into proper alignment, muscle engagement, and breath awareness to help you optimize your practice and avoid potential pitfalls.

7. **Practice Consistently**: Consistency is key to refining your technique and form in face yoga. Commit to practicing regularly and incorporate feedback from your instructor or personal observations to continually refine and improve your skills. Set aside dedicated time for practice each day or week and prioritize self-care and mindfulness in your routine.

By fine-tuning your technique and form in face yoga, you can maximize the benefits of your practice, minimize the risk of injury, and cultivate a deeper connection with your body and breath. Focus on alignment, mindful muscle engagement, controlled movement, breath awareness, and modification as needed to refine your practice and achieve optimal results over time.

6.3 Avoiding Common Mistakes

Avoiding common mistakes in face yoga can help you maximize the effectiveness of your practice and minimize the risk of injury. Here are some tips for identifying and avoiding common pitfalls:

1. **Overexertion**: Avoid overexerting yourself during face yoga exercises, as this can lead to muscle strain or fatigue. Start gradually and listen to your body's feedback, stopping if you experience any pain or discomfort. Progress at a pace that feels comfortable and sustainable for you.

2. **Poor Posture**: Maintain proper posture throughout your practice to support stability and alignment. Avoid slouching or rounding your back, and keep your shoulders relaxed and away from your ears.

Engage your core muscles to support your spine and maintain a neutral position.

3. **Excessive Tension**: Be mindful of tension in your face and neck muscles during exercises. While some degree of muscle engagement is necessary for effective practice, avoid excessive tension or straining. Focus on using the appropriate muscles for each exercise and relax any unnecessary tension.

4. **Ignoring Breath**: Neglecting to coordinate your breath with your movements can detract from the effectiveness and mindfulness of your practice. Remember to breathe deeply and rhythmically throughout your practice, using your breath to facilitate relaxation, deepen stretches, and enhance muscle engagement.

5. **Lack of Variation**: Avoid sticking to the same exercises or routines without incorporating variation.

Including a variety of exercises that target different muscle groups can prevent plateauing and keep your practice engaging and effective. Experiment with new techniques and challenges to continually challenge your muscles and promote growth.

6. **Skipping Warm-Up and Cool-Down**: Skipping warm-up and cool-down exercises can increase the risk of injury and decrease the effectiveness of your practice. Take the time to properly warm up your muscles before engaging in more intense exercises, and conclude your practice with relaxation and stretching to promote recovery and relaxation.

7. **Pushing Through Pain**: Ignoring pain or discomfort during face yoga exercises can lead to injury or exacerbate existing issues. If you experience any pain or discomfort, stop the exercise immediately and assess the situation. Modify the exercise as needed or consult a

qualified instructor or healthcare professional for guidance.

8. **Expecting Immediate Results**: Face yoga, like any form of exercise, requires time, consistency, and patience to yield noticeable results. Avoid expecting immediate or drastic changes and instead focus on the process of practice and gradual improvement over time. Celebrate small victories and milestones along the way, knowing that consistent effort will lead to lasting results.

Avoiding common mistakes and practicing mindfully, you can enhance the effectiveness and safety of your face yoga practice, minimize the risk of injury, and maximize the benefits for your physical and mental well-being. Prioritize proper technique, mindfulness, and self-awareness in your practice, and enjoy the journey of self-discovery and transformation.

CHAPTER 7

Incorporating Mindfulness and Meditation

7.1 Mind-Body Connection in Face Yoga

Incorporating mindfulness and meditation into your face yoga practice can deepen your awareness of the mind-body connection, enhance relaxation, and promote overall well-being. Here's how you can cultivate a deeper mind-body connection in your face yoga practice:

1. **Present-Moment Awareness**: Practice being fully present in the moment during your face yoga practice. Instead of allowing your mind to wander or dwell on past or future concerns, focus your attention on the sensations in your body as you perform each exercise. Notice the subtle movements of your facial muscles, the rhythm of your breath, and the quality of your thoughts and emotions.

2. **Body Scan Meditation**: Begin your face yoga practice with a body scan meditation to cultivate awareness of tension, discomfort, or areas of imbalance in your body. Start at the top of your head and gradually scan down through your body, bringing attention to each area and noticing any sensations that arise. Pay special attention to your face, jaw, and neck, releasing any tension or holding patterns as you become aware of them.

3. **Breath Awareness**: Use your breath as an anchor for mindfulness throughout your face yoga practice. Focus on the sensations of the breath as it enters and leaves your body, observing the rise and fall of your chest and abdomen with each inhale and exhale. Use deep, diaphragmatic breathing to promote relaxation and presence, allowing your breath to guide you deeper into each movement and stretch.

4. **Mindful Movement**: Perform each face yoga exercise with mindfulness and intention, focusing on the quality of your movements rather than rushing through the motions. Notice the sensations in your facial muscles as you engage them, and observe any thoughts or emotions that arise without judgment. Cultivate a sense of curiosity and openness as you explore the connections between your mind and body.

5. **Body Awareness**: Develop greater body awareness through your face

yoga practice by tuning into the signals and feedback that your body provides. Notice any areas of tension, discomfort, or resistance, and adjust your practice accordingly to honor your body's needs and limitations. Pay attention to how different movements and exercises affect your body and mind, and adapt your practice as needed to promote balance and harmony.

6. **Gratitude and Intention Setting**: Cultivate an attitude of gratitude and set positive intentions for your face yoga practice. Begin each session by expressing gratitude for your body and the opportunity to nurture your physical and mental well-being through practice. Set an intention or dedication for your practice, such as cultivating self-love, promoting relaxation, or embracing inner peace.

7. **Integration with Meditation Practices**: Incorporate meditation practices such as loving-kindness meditation, body scan meditation, or

mindfulness of breath into your face yoga routine to deepen your mindfulness and relaxation. Dedicate time at the end of your practice to sit in silent meditation, allowing yourself to bask in the afterglow of your practice and integrate the benefits of mindfulness into your daily life.

cultivating a deeper mind-body connection in your face yoga practice, you can enhance the effectiveness of your exercises, promote relaxation and stress relief, and cultivate greater overall well-being. Embrace mindfulness and meditation as integral components of your face yoga routine, and enjoy the transformative journey of self-discovery and self-care.

7.2 Meditation Techniques for Facial Relaxation

Incorporating meditation techniques into your face yoga practice can help promote deep relaxation and release tension in the facial muscles. Here are some meditation techniques specifically designed for facial relaxation:

1. **Body Scan Meditation**: Begin by finding a comfortable seated or lying position with your spine straight and your body relaxed. Close your eyes and bring your awareness to your breath. Take a few deep breaths to center yourself. Start at the top of your head and slowly scan down through your body, bringing attention to cach arca and consciously releasing tension as you go. When you reach your face, focus on softening the muscles of your forehead, eyes, cheeks, jaw, and neck. Visualize any tension melting away with each exhale, leaving your face feeling relaxed and at ease.

2. **Progressive Muscle Relaxation**: Sit or lie down in a comfortable position and close your eyes. Begin by tensing the muscles in your forehead by scrunching up your eyebrows and holding for a few seconds, then

release and allow the muscles to relax completely. Move on to the muscles around your eyes, cheeks, jaw, and neck, tensing each muscle group for a few seconds before releasing. Focus on the sensation of relaxation spreading throughout your face and neck with each release, allowing any remaining tension to dissolve away.

3. **Breath Awareness Meditation**: Sit comfortably and close your eyes. Bring your awareness to your breath as it moves in and out of your body. Notice the sensation of the breath as it enters and leaves your nostrils, fills your lungs, and expands your chest and abdomen. With each exhale, imagine any tension in your face melting away, leaving behind a sense of calm and relaxation. Continue to focus on your breath, using it as an anchor to keep your mind present and centered.

4. **Visualizing a Relaxing Scene**: Close your eyes and take a few deep

breaths to relax your body and mind. Visualize yourself in a peaceful and serene environment, such as a tranquil beach, a lush forest, or a serene mountaintop. Picture yourself surrounded by beauty and tranquility, feeling the warmth of the sun on your skin and the gentle breeze on your face. Allow yourself to fully immerse in this visualization, experiencing a deep sense of relaxation and ease.

5. **Affirmation Meditation**: Choose a positive affirmation related to relaxation and facial harmony, such as "My face is relaxed and at ease," or "I release tension from my facial muscles with each breath." Close your eyes and repeat the affirmation silently or aloud, allowing its meaning to sink in with each repetition. Visualize the affirmation as true in your mind's eye, feeling the relaxation and ease spreading throughout your face and body with each repetition.

These meditation techniques into your face yoga practice, you can enhance relaxation, release tension in the facial muscles, and promote overall well-being. Experiment with different techniques to find what works best for you, and enjoy the rejuvenating benefits of a relaxed and harmonious face and mind.

CHAPTER 8

Maintaining Results and Long-Term Benefits

8.1 Consistency and Persistence

Consistency and persistence are key factors in maintaining the results and long-term benefits of your face yoga practice. Here's why they are essential and how you can incorporate them into your routine:

1. **Muscle Memory**: Just like any form of exercise, consistent practice of face yoga helps build muscle

memory. By repeatedly engaging and strengthening the facial muscles through targeted exercises, you reinforce the desired muscle tone and contour, which contributes to long-term improvements in facial appearance.

2. **Preventing Muscle Atrophy**: Regular face yoga practice helps prevent muscle atrophy, which can occur due to aging or lack of use. By consistently engaging and exercising the facial muscles, you promote circulation, oxygenation, and nutrient delivery to the tissues, which can help maintain muscle tone and prevent sagging or drooping over time.

3. **Progressive Improvement**: Consistent practice allows you to gradually progress and improve in your face yoga journey. As you continue to practice regularly, you may notice subtle but cumulative changes in your facial appearance, muscle tone, and overall well-being.

These improvements build upon each other over time, leading to more significant and sustainable results in the long run.

4. **Integration into Daily Routine**: Incorporating face yoga into your daily routine helps make it a habit and ensures that you consistently allocate time for practice. Whether you practice in the morning, during breaks throughout the day, or as part of your evening wind-down routine, find a time that works best for you and commit to it consistently.

5. **Mindfulness and Awareness**: Consistent practice fosters mindfulness and awareness of your facial muscles and expressions throughout the day. By regularly engaging in face yoga exercises, you become more attuned to facial tension, stress, or habits that may contribute to wrinkles or asymmetry. This heightened awareness allows you to make conscious adjustments

and maintain the benefits of your practice over time.

6. **Long-Term Health and Well-Being**: Beyond aesthetic improvements, consistent face yoga practice contributes to long-term health and well-being. By promoting relaxation, reducing stress, and enhancing circulation, face yoga supports overall skin health, collagen production, and cellular regeneration, which can contribute to a more youthful and radiant complexion over time.

To incorporate consistency and persistence into your face yoga practice, consider the following tips:

- **Set Realistic Goals**: Establish achievable goals for your face yoga practice, taking into account your schedule, lifestyle, and personal preferences. Break down larger goals into smaller milestones and celebrate your progress along the way.

- **Create a Routine**: Develop a consistent routine for your face yoga practice, incorporating it into your daily or weekly schedule like any other self-care activity. Set aside dedicated time for practice and prioritize it as an essential part of your wellness routine.

- **Track Your Progress**: Keep track of your progress and achievements in your face yoga journey. Take photos or journal about your experiences, noting any changes in facial appearance, muscle tone, or overall well-being over time. Reflect on your journey and celebrate your successes.

- **Stay Motivated**: Stay motivated and inspired by experimenting with new exercises, techniques, or challenges in your face yoga practice. Connect with a supportive community of fellow practitioners or seek guidance from qualified instructors to stay engaged and motivated on your journey.

- **Practice Self-Compassion**: Be kind and compassionate with yourself on your face yoga journey. Embrace the ups and downs, and remember that progress takes time and patience. Treat yourself with love and understanding, and trust in the process as you work towards your goals.

Prioritizing consistency and persistence in your face yoga practice, you can maintain the results and long-term benefits of your efforts, leading to a healthier, happier, and more radiant you.

8.2 Lifestyle Factors for Facial Health

Maintaining facial health goes beyond just practicing face yoga. Several lifestyle factors can significantly impact the health and appearance of your skin and facial muscles. Here are some lifestyle habits that can contribute to facial health:

1. **Healthy Diet**: A balanced and nutritious diet plays a crucial role in supporting overall skin health. Incorporate plenty of fruits, vegetables, lean proteins, and whole grains into your diet to provide essential vitamins, minerals, and antioxidants that promote skin elasticity, collagen production, and cellular repair.

2. **Hydration**: Proper hydration is essential for maintaining skin elasticity and hydration. Drink plenty of water throughout the day to keep your skin hydrated and plump. Limit consumption of dehydrating beverages such as alcohol and caffeine, which can contribute to dryness and dullness.

3. **Sun Protection**: Protecting your skin from harmful UV rays is essential for preventing premature aging and damage. Apply a broad-spectrum sunscreen with an SPF of 30 or higher daily, even on cloudy days, and wear protective clothing and

accessories such as hats and sunglasses when outdoors.

4. **Skincare Routine**: Establishing a consistent skincare routine tailored to your skin type and concerns can help keep your skin healthy and radiant. Cleanse, moisturize, and protect your skin daily, and incorporate additional treatments such as exfoliation, serums, and masks as needed to address specific concerns.

5. **Stress Management**: Chronic stress can negatively impact skin health by triggering inflammation, breakouts, and premature aging. Practice stress-reducing techniques such as meditation, deep breathing, yoga, or mindfulness to promote relaxation and balance in your life.

6. **Quality Sleep**: Adequate sleep is essential for skin regeneration and repair. Aim for 7-9 hours of quality sleep per night to allow your skin cells to rejuvenate and replenish. Invest in a comfortable mattress and

pillows and establish a relaxing bedtime routine to promote restful sleep.

7. **Facial Exercises**: In addition to face yoga, incorporate facial exercises into your routine to strengthen and tone facial muscles. Facial exercises can help improve muscle definition, lift sagging skin, and enhance overall facial appearance when performed regularly.

8. **Smoking Cessation**: Smoking accelerates skin aging by reducing blood flow, depleting collagen levels, and causing oxidative stress. If you smoke, consider quitting to improve skin health and prevent premature wrinkles and fine lines.

9. **Limiting Alcohol and Caffeine**: Excessive alcohol and caffeine consumption can dehydrate the skin and contribute to inflammation and puffiness. Limit your intake of alcoholic and caffeinated beverages

and opt for water, herbal tea, or green juice instead.

10. **Regular Exercise**: Regular exercise promotes circulation, oxygenation, and detoxification, which are essential for healthy skin. Incorporate cardiovascular exercise, strength training, and flexibility exercises into your routine to support overall health and vitality.

Adopting these lifestyle factors for facial health in conjunction with your face yoga practice, you can maximize the benefits and maintain long-term results for a healthy, radiant complexion.

8.3 Adapting Your Practice Over Time

As you progress in your face yoga journey and experience changes in your body, lifestyle, and goals, it's important to adapt your practice to suit your evolving needs. Here are some tips for adapting your face yoga practice over time:

1. **Assess Your Goals**: Regularly reassess your goals and objectives for practicing face yoga. Consider whether your goals have shifted, if you've achieved your initial targets, or if new concerns have emerged that you'd like to address. Adjust your practice accordingly to align with your current aspirations and priorities.

2. **Evaluate Your Progress**: Take time to evaluate your progress and results from your face yoga practice. Assess any changes in your facial appearance, muscle tone, and overall well-being, and consider whether your current routine is effectively meeting your needs. Reflect on what has worked well for you and what areas could benefit from adjustment or refinement.

3. **Explore New Techniques**: Keep your practice fresh and engaging by exploring new face yoga techniques, exercises, or variations. Experiment with different movements,

sequences, or challenges to target specific muscle groups, address new concerns, or add variety to your routine. Stay open to learning and growth as you continue to evolve in your practice.

4. **Modify Intensity and Duration**: Adjust the intensity and duration of your face yoga practice based on your energy levels, schedule, and personal preferences. If you're feeling fatigued or overwhelmed, consider scaling back the intensity or duration of your practice to prevent burnout and promote sustainability. Conversely, if you're feeling energized and motivated, challenge yourself with longer sessions or more advanced exercises.

5. **Listen to Your Body**: Tune into your body's feedback and listen to its signals during your face yoga practice. Pay attention to any sensations of discomfort, tension, or strain, and modify or adapt your practice as needed to honor your

body's needs and limitations. Avoid pushing through pain or overexerting yourself, and prioritize self-care and self-compassion in your practice.

6. **Seek Guidance as Needed**: Don't hesitate to seek guidance from qualified instructors, practitioners, or healthcare professionals if you encounter challenges or have questions about your face yoga practice. A skilled instructor can offer personalized advice, modifications, and support to help you navigate your practice and achieve your goals effectively.

8.4 Embracing the Journey of Face Yoga

Embracing the journey of face yoga involves cultivating a mindset of self-discovery, self-care, and personal growth as you engage in this transformative practice. Here are some ways to embrace the journey of face yoga:

1. **Cultivate Self-Acceptance**: Embrace your unique features and facial expressions with love and acceptance. Recognize that beauty comes in many forms and that imperfections are a natural part of being human. Practice self-compassion and celebrate your individuality as you embark on your face yoga journey.

2. **Focus on Inner Beauty**: While face yoga can enhance external appearance, remember that true beauty radiates from within. Cultivate inner beauty through qualities such as kindness, compassion, gratitude, and authenticity. Nurture your inner landscape with mindfulness practices, positive affirmations, and acts of self-love and kindness.

3. **Celebrate Progress, Not Perfection**: Shift your focus from achieving perfection to celebrating progress and growth. Recognize and celebrate the small victories and

milestones along your face yoga journey, whether it's noticing subtle improvements in muscle tone, feeling more relaxed and rejuvenated, or experiencing increased self-confidence and self-awareness.

4. **Embrace the Process**: Embrace the process of learning and growth inherent in your face yoga practice. View each practice session as an opportunity for self-discovery, exploration, and refinement. Embrace the ups and downs, challenges and triumphs, and moments of stillness and movement as integral parts of your journey.

5. **Stay Curious and Open-Minded**: Approach your face yoga practice with curiosity and an open mind. Explore different techniques, exercises, and approaches to discover what resonates with you and supports your unique needs and goals. Stay open to learning from others, trying new things, and

adapting your practice over time as you evolve.

6. **Practice Gratitude**: Cultivate an attitude of gratitude for the opportunity to engage in face yoga and nurture your facial health and well-being. Express gratitude for your body, your breath, and the ability to care for yourself through practice. Incorporate gratitude practices into your routine, such as keeping a gratitude journal or offering thanks before and after each practice session.

7. **Connect with Community**: Seek support and connection from a community of fellow face yoga practitioners. Share your experiences, challenges, and insights with others who are on a similar journey. Draw inspiration from their stories, offer encouragement and support, and celebrate each other's progress and achievements.

8. **Listen to Your Intuition**: Trust your intuition and inner wisdom as you navigate your face yoga journey. Tune into your body's signals, feelings, and sensations during practice, and honor what feels right for you. Allow your intuition to guide you in making decisions about your practice, whether it's choosing exercises, setting intentions, or adapting your routine.

9. **Be Patient and Persistent**: Embrace patience and persistence as you progress in your face yoga practice. Recognize that change takes time and that results may not be immediate. Stay committed to your practice, even on days when motivation wanes or progress feels slow. Trust in the process and believe in the power of consistent effort and dedication to bring about transformation over time.

10. **Find Joy and Fulfillment**: Above all, find joy and fulfillment in your face yoga practice. Let it be a source

of pleasure, rejuvenation, and self-expression in your life. Infuse your practice with elements that bring you joy, whether it's listening to uplifting music, practicing in nature, or simply smiling and laughing as you engage with your facial muscles.

By embracing the journey of face yoga with self-acceptance, mindfulness, gratitude, and persistence, you can cultivate a deeper connection with yourself, enhance your facial health and well-being, and experience greater joy and fulfillment along the way. Enjoy the transformative journey of self-discovery and self-care as you embark on your face yoga journey.

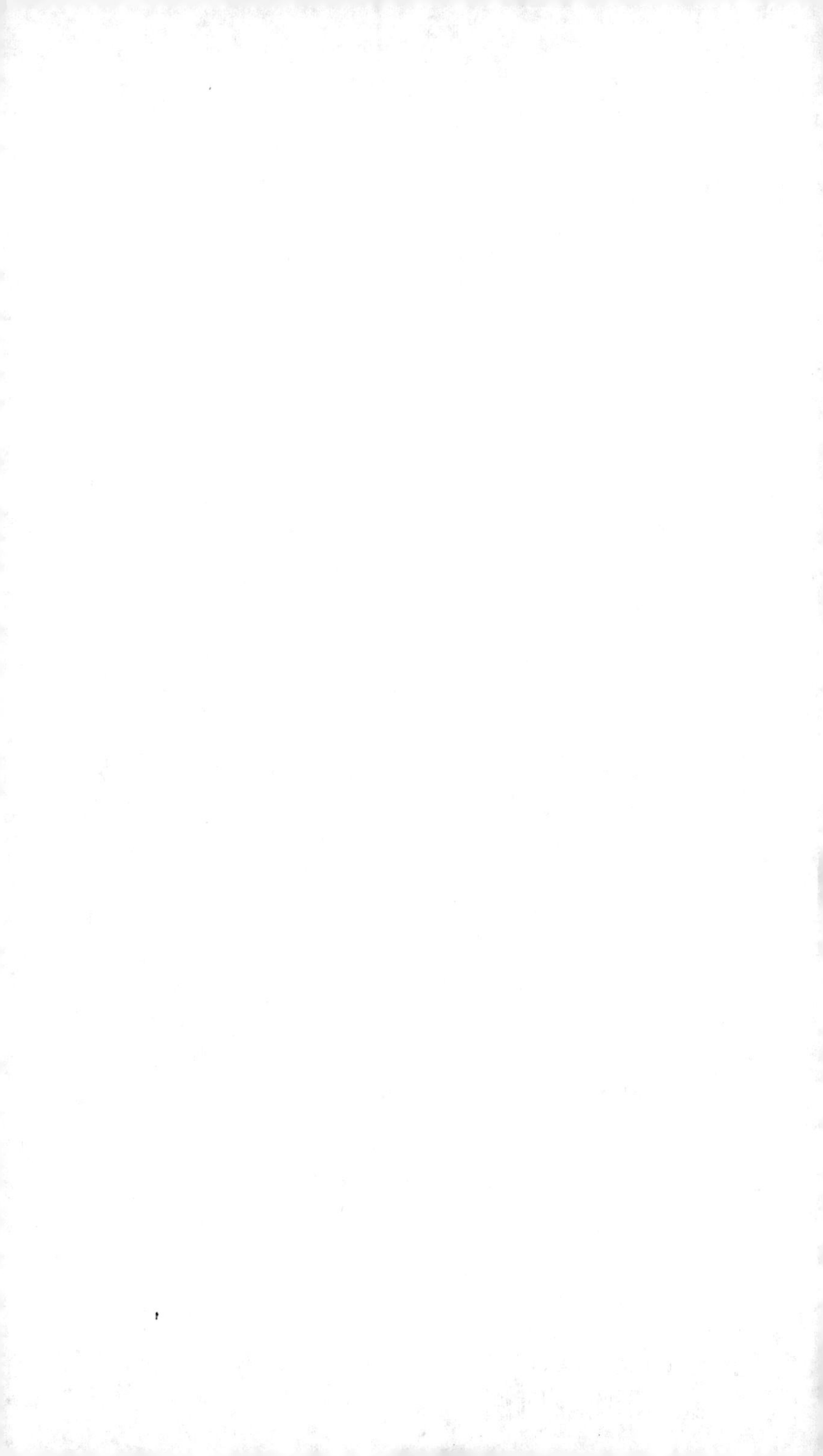